The Holistic Pet Care Guide

Natural Wellness for Cats & Dogs

Steph. Gamelin

Disclaimer

The information provided in this book is for educational and informational purposes only. It is not intended as medical or veterinary advice. The author and publisher do not accept any responsibility for any liability, loss or risk, personal or otherwise, incurred as a consequence, directly or indirectly, from the use and application of any of the suggestions, preparations, or procedures in this book. Readers need to regularly consult a physician or veterinarian in matters relating to their health, pet's health, particularly if any symptoms that may require diagnosis or medical attention occur. It is the reader's sole responsibility to discuss and verify any information obtained from this book with a licensed veterinarian concerning the pet's specific condition. Always seek the advice of your veterinarian or other qualified veterinary provider before using any supplements or herbal remedies with your pet.

The recipes and formula preparation instructions described in this book have been formulated with care and are believed to be nutritious and beneficial based on the ingredients used. However, the reader is cautioned to use judgment when administering homemade supplements and herbal remedies.

This book does not recommend ignoring conventional medical advice or delaying seeking it due to information provided herein. This book does not make any promises or guarantees regarding results obtained from using the remedies outlined herein. Individual results may vary.

In no event shall the author be liable for any direct, indirect, consequential, special, exemplary, or other damages arising from the use or misuse of any formulas, preparations, or information contained in this book.

The information presented herein represents the views of the author as of the date of publication. The information contained herein is subject to change without notice.

Please consult with your veterinarian or other qualified healthcare provider before using any herbal remedies or supplements mentioned in this book. Proper veterinarian oversight is essential.

CONTENTS

Introduction

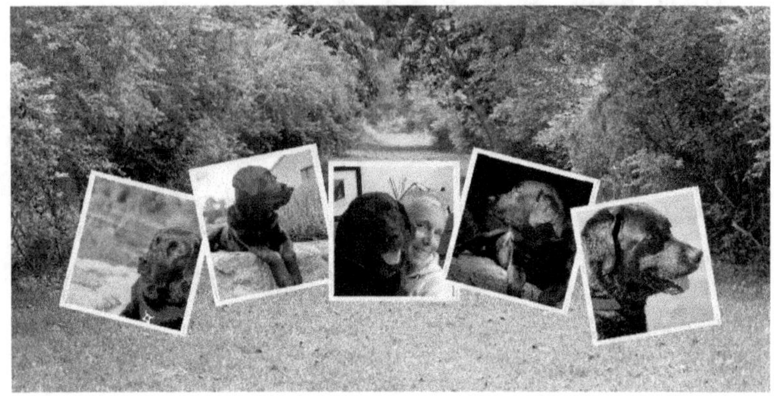

My journey towards holistic pet care began nine years ago, when I adopted my beloved Labrador Retriever, Jamba.

She was 11 months old when I picked her up from the breeder, but unfortunately, was not in good condition. Jamba had severe ear infections in both ears, resulting in painful otitis. She also had visible skin parasites and was underweight for her age. I immediately brought her to the vet, where we discovered she had intestinal parasites as well. My heart broke to see this sweet pup suffering from preventable issues at such a young age.

After putting Jamba on medications to clear up the infections and parasites, I was relieved she quickly rebounded into a happy, energetic dog. We bonded instantly, cherishing our evenings snuggling on the couch and mornings spent playing fetch in the yard. Jamba could keep up on hikes through the woods and never turned away from a game of catch. She enjoyed robust health as a young dog.

When Jamba turned eight, I began noticing subtle changes. She no longer leapt as nimbly up the stairs. Our walks slowed down as she started lagging behind to rest. At age ten, Jamba developed digestive issues that left her gassy and occasionally vomiting. Then the chronic ear infections returned, likely tied to allergies. My once energetic pup was slowly becoming lethargic and uncomfortable.

Seeing Jamba struggle with these age-related health problems broke my heart. The vet prescribed anti-inflammatories and special food, but they only provided minimal relief. I knew many aging dogs developed arthritis and other issues, but it pained me to see those early in Jamba...

Having researched holistic health for my own needs, I knew there were many gentle herbal remedies that could support dogs.

With vet approval, I started supplementing Jamba's diet with turmeric, fish oil, and boswellia to reduce inflammation and arthritis. Within weeks she had more energy and no longer hesitated to jump in the car. I also gave Jamba chamomile tea to relax her during thunderstorms that previously stressed her out. These early successes using natural supplements motivated me to learn more.

In this book, I want to share everything I've discovered about herbal remedies for common pet issues like joint pain, digestion, anxiety, liver health and more. I aim to provide pet owners like myself with guidance, recipes, and resources to improve their furry friends' health and avoid prescription medication side effects when possible. Let's start exploring nature's solutions for our pets' wellbeing!

Chapter 1

Herbs for Reducing Inflammation

and Joint Pain

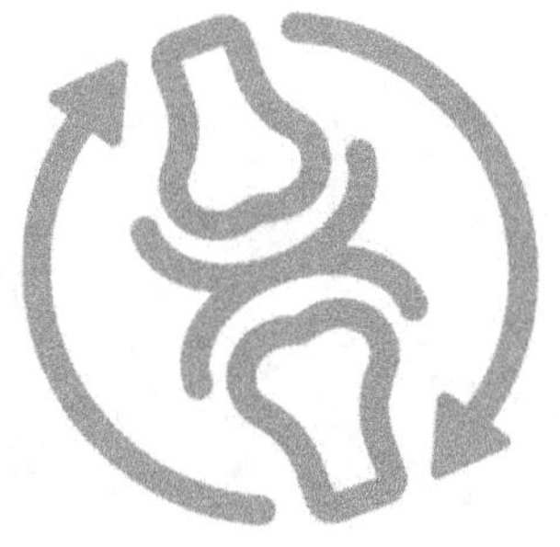

Introduction

Arthritis and joint pain are unfortunately common issues for aging pets. Over half of dogs over the age of seven have arthritis, which can seriously impact their mobility and quality of life.

Cats can also suffer from stiff, inflamed joints as they get older. Seeing our furry companions struggle to get up and down or limp around the house is heartbreaking. While prescription anti-inflammatories and pain medications are an option, they can have concerning side effects with long-term use.

The good news is there are many natural supplements that can help reduce inflammation, stiffness, and discomfort in pets with arthritis or joint injuries.

In this chapter we'll explore the top anti-inflammatory herbs for pets and how to safely administer them. The goal is keeping pets active and improving their mobility without relying solely on medications.

I. Turmeric

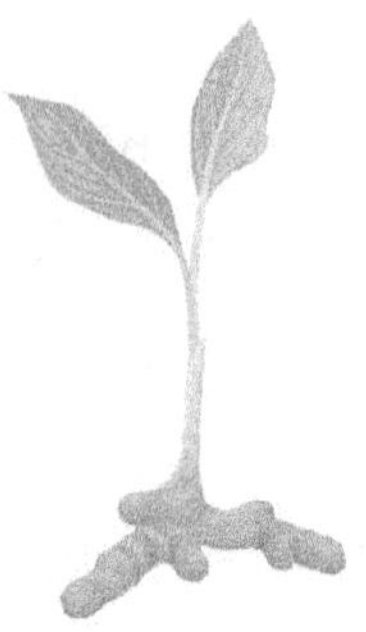

Turmeric is likely the most popular herbal anti-inflammatory, thanks to its active compound curcumin. Curcumin has been found in studies to reduce levels of inflammation-causing enzymes in the body.

Turmeric can provide similar pain and inflammation relief as NSAID medications without the high risk of gastrointestinal side effects.

Furthermore, it serves as an antioxidant to neutralize free radicals and may even help protect joints from additional damage. Numerous veterinarians and pet health experts recommend turmeric for dogs with arthritis.

The typical dosage is 15-20 mg per pound of body weight per day, either split into two doses or given all at once.

Turmeric should be administered with food for optimal absorption.

Potential side effects to monitor include diarrhea and vomiting if the dosage is too high. Combining turmeric with piperine (black pepper extract) can boost absorption substantially.

Overall, **turmeric is an excellent herbal option for managing chronic inflammatory issues in pets like arthritis.**

II. CBD Oil

CBD, or cannabidiol oil, has become very popular for treating pain, arthritis, seizures, and other health problems in dogs and cats.

Unlike THC found in marijuana, CBD does not produce any psychoactive effects but still provides powerful therapeutic benefits. CBD acts on the endocannabinoid system to reduce the sensation of pain and minimize inflammation.

Multiple studies have shown CBD oil can improve mobility and comfort in dogs with osteoarthritis.

The optimal dosage varies based on the size of your pet and severity of symptoms. A typical starting amount is 0.5 - 2 mg per pound administered twice daily. It's best to consult with a holistic veterinarian for specific dosage recommendations.

High quality CBD manufactured specifically for pets is essential for safety, as unregulated products may contain toxic ingredients. Potential side effects can include dry mouth, drowsiness, or gastrointestinal upset.

Monitoring your pet's reaction is important when first starting CBD oil.

III. Boswellia

Boswellia is an Ayurvedic herb derived from the Boswellia serrata tree in India. The active compounds are boswellic acids that provide potent anti-inflammatory and analgesic effects.

Research on boswellia for dogs suggests it can significantly improve mobility, stiffness, and pain associated with arthritis and other joint issues.

For cats it also helps reduce inflammation from arthritis and injuries.

The typical dosage for boswellia is 75-100 mg per day for every 10 pounds of body weight. Look for formulas standardized to contain 60-65% boswellic acids for optimal potency.

Boswellia is safe for long-term use and has minimal side effects, though it can cause digestive upset on an empty stomach. It is often combined with glucosamine/chondroitin supplements or turmeric for additional joint support.

IV. Other Anti-Inflammatory Herbs

There are a few other beneficial anti-inflammatory herbs for pets including ginger, devil's claw, yucca, and celery seed.

Ginger contains active compounds called gingerols that reduce inflammation. The dosage is 1/8 teaspoon powdered ginger per 20 pounds of body weight twice daily.

Devil's claw is an African herb used for centuries to treat arthritis and back pain.

Yucca also helps with joint pain and stiffness through its steroid-like saponins.

Celery seed supports joint health through its antioxidant and anti-inflammatory properties.

These can all be rotated or combined with the main supplements above. Always verify dosing guidelines and monitor for side effects like digestion upset.

Below is a summary table of the main joint health herbs, forms, and recommended dosages:

Herb	Form	Dosage - Small Dogs	Dosage - Large Dogs	Frequency
Turmeric	Powder, capsules	15-20 mg	25-40 mg	Daily or every other day
CBD oil	Oil, treats	0.5-2 mg per lb	1-2 mg per lb	Twice daily
Boswellia	Capsules, chews	75-100 mg per 10 lbs	100-150 mg per 10 lbs	Daily
Ginger	Powder, capsules	125-250 mg	500-1000 mg	Twice daily as needed

V. Lifestyle Changes

While herbal supplements are very helpful for managing arthritis and joint pain, making some lifestyle changes can provide additional benefits:

- Encouraging weight loss if your pet is overweight to reduce strain on joints
- Providing ramps, orthopedic beds, and easy access to food/water
- Joint-supportive diets rich in omega-3s and antioxidants
- Low-impact exercise like short walks, swimming, or massage therapy
- Alternative treatments like acupuncture, laser therapy, stem cell therapy

Keeping your arthritic pet active and at a healthy weight are key to maximizing their comfort and mobility. The remedies in this chapter can make a big difference in easing inflammation and pain. Always consult your veterinarian before starting any new supplements. Together you can give your beloved pet a better quality of life as they age.

Chapter 2

Herbs for Calming Pet Anxiety

Introduction

Pet anxiety is on the rise, with some estimates stating 15-20% of dogs and cats suffer from various anxiety disorders.

Anxiety can manifest in pets as furniture scratching, urinating/defecating indoors, hiding, aggression, obsessive behaviors, and more.

The causes range from trauma, abuse, neglect, phobias, separation anxiety, and changes in environment or routine.

Pets may also experience social stress around other animals or people.

While behavioral and pharmaceutical treatments are options, herbal remedies can provide gentle anxiety relief without sedation or side effects.

Certain herbs interact with pet neurotransmitters like GABA to reduce excitability and promote relaxation.

This chapter will explore the top herbs for relieving anxiety and helping stressed pets feel more calm and comfortable.

I. Valerian

Sophie's Journey to Calmness

> *Sophie, a spirited Border Collie, had always been prone to anxiety, especially during thunderstorms. Her owner, Emily, tried various remedies with minimal success until she discovered valerian root. Emily shares, "Valerian became Sophie's saving grace. During storms, I'd give her a valerian supplement, and she'd lie calmly by my side, unaffected by the thunder and lightning. It was like a miracle."*
> *Sophie's story is a testament to the power of valerian in soothing anxious pets during stressful situations.*

Valerian root is one of the most validated herbal sedatives used for centuries to promote sleep and relaxation.

The active components like valerenic acid and valepotriates interact with GABA and serotonin receptors responsible for calming the central nervous system.

Multiple studies have shown valerian can reduce anxiety-related behaviors and restlessness in dogs.

For noise phobia such as during thunderstorms or fireworks, valerian helped 70% of treated dogs significantly based on owner surveys.

The dosage for dogs is 1-2 mg powdered valerian root per pound of body weight given 1-3 times per day.

For cats, the dosage is 1/4-1/2 tablet or capsule twice daily.

Monitor for potential side effects like gastrointestinal upset, drowsiness, or agitation if the dose is too high.

II. Chamomile

Chamomile's Gentle Touch

> *Luna, a sweet-natured Persian cat, often struggled with nervousness when meeting new people. Her owner, Mark, decided to try chamomile tea as a calming solution.*
> *"Adding a bit of chamomile tea to Luna's water bowl before guests arrived made a remarkable difference," Mark explains.*
> *"She remained serene and content, transforming her once-anxious demeanor into one of quiet confidence."*

The daisy-like flowers of German chamomile contain medicinal compounds proven to reduce anxiety and calm restlessness in pets. Chamomile has mild sedative effects to relieve stress while also promoting gut health and soothing skin irritations sometimes worsened by anxiety.

For anxious dogs, administer 3-4 cups of cooled chamomile tea per day added to food or water.

Cats can have 1-2 tablespoons daily added to a meal. Chamomile tinctures or liquid extracts at dosages of 1-3 mL per day are another option.

Always source food-grade chamomile tea and high quality extracts to prevent toxicity issues from contamination. Observe for potential mild diarrhea or drowsiness.

III. Passionflower

Passionflower has a long history of use among Native Americans for promoting relaxation and sleep. Today it is still used for anxiety, nerves, and insomnia.

The flavonoids in passionflower have anticonvulsant, sedative, and anti-anxiety effects.
For dogs, the dosage is 1/4 to 1/2 dropperful of passionflower tincture per 25 pounds of body weight. It can be added to food or water twice daily.

Cats can have 1/4 dropperful twice a day. Look for high quality tinctures with consistent dosing of passionflower aerial parts.

Monitor for potential side effects like inhibition of MAOIs and blood thinners when combining with other medications.

IV. Other Calming Herbs

Certain other herbs can provide anxiety relief for pets, such as CBD oil, catnip, lemon balm, and skullcap.

CBD interacts with endocannabinoid receptors involved in mood, pain perception, and more.

Catnip contains nepetalactone that induces sedation in cats but not dogs.

Lemon balm and skullcap also have anti-anxiety components. Lemon balm helps your dog feel more relaxed, soothing stress and encouraging calmer behavior.

These can be rotated or combined in formulas with the herbs above for added benefits.

Always verify safety and dosing when using new herbs or combinations.

Herbalist Karen R.

Karen R., an experienced herbalist dedicated to pet wellness, shares her perspective.

"The synergy between herbs and pet well-being is profound," says Karen. "Herbs like chamomile and passionflower have a centuries-old history of calming both body and mind. When used correctly, they can provide profound comfort to our beloved pets, allowing them to lead happier, more relaxed lives."

Below is a chart summarizing common anti-anxiety herbs, their forms, and dosage ranges:

Herb	Form	Dosage - Small Dogs	Dosage - Large Dogs
Valerian	Powdered root	1-2 mg per lb	1-2 mg per lb
Chamomile	Tea, tincture	3-4 cups tea per day	3-4 cups tea per day
Passionflower	Tincture	1/4-1/2 dropper per 25 lbs	1/2-1 dropper per 25 lbs
CBD Oil	Oil, treats	0.5-2 mg per lb	1-2 mg per lb

V. Lifestyle Changes

While herbal supplementation can help greatly with pet anxiety, making changes to your home and routines can provide additional benefits:

- Ensuring your pet has a dedicated safe space or crate for retreat
- Diffusing calming pheromones
- Sticking to a consistent daily schedule
- Training techniques to reinforce desired calm behaviors
- Exercising and playing with pets to release energy
- Working with your vet on anti-anxiety medication if needed

With some patience helping anxious pets adjust, herbal remedies can promote relaxation, reduce chronic stress, and improve your pet's overall wellbeing. The therapies in this chapter can make a big difference in easing an anxious pet's mind and body.

Chapter 3

Supporting Digestion and Gut Health

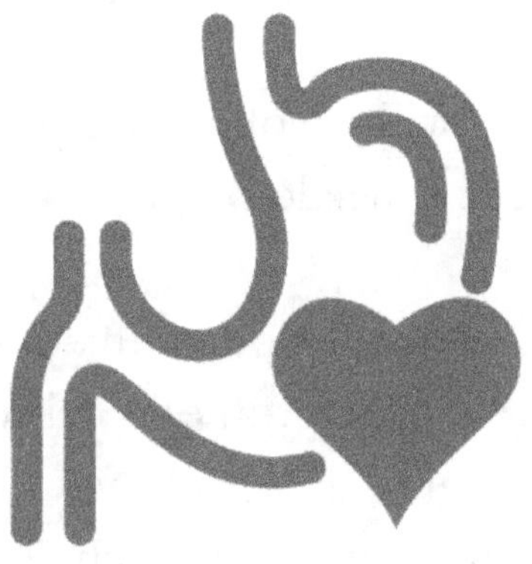

When I first adopted my Labrador Retriever puppy Jamba, I fed her a popular commercial dry dog food that was conveniently available at all the grocery and pet stores.

However, I quickly noticed that she had recurrent gas, loose stools, and vomiting. Jamba just didn't seem to tolerate the processed kibble well.

I started researching and learned how dry pet foods are highly processed, contain synthetic additives, and lack nutrients that support healthy digestion.

Many pet owners don't realize the toll that conventional diets can take on a dog or cat's gastrointestinal system over time. Signs like inflammatory bowel disease, colitis, chronic vomiting, diarrhea, and gas are rampant in pets these days.

There are even risks of disease from contamination. Improving digestion can also boost immunity, nutrient absorption, and overall well being.

That's why I transitioned Jamba to a more natural, species-appropriate diet and started using several herbal remedies to get her gut health back on track.

In this chapter, we'll explore my top botanical picks for optimizing pet digestion and soothing gastrointestinal issues. Slippery elm, marshmallow root, papaya, ginger, and probiotics have worked wonders for Jamba's tummy.

I'll share how each one works, proper dosing, administration tips, and the lifestyle changes that provide additional benefits. Give your furry friend the relief they deserve and get their digestive system functioning optimally.

Introduction

As they are famous for their unquenchable appetite, it's not uncommon for a dog to suffer from indigestion or stomach issues. Canine stomach ache is usually a result of spoiled food, a food intolerance or allergy, or because they have ingested something questionable.

Most tummy issues are easily treated by the vet, but if you'd like to alleviate your pup's pain naturally at home, check out the following herbal remedies and advice.

What usually causes an upset stomach in dogs?

Although dogs can suffer from severe digestive problems, if your furry friend has symptoms of an upset stomach, it's most probably because he ingested something he wasn't supposed to.

Vomiting, bloating, diarrhea, and pain are just the body's fighting mechanisms to deal with the gut imposter.

Another common reason for an upset stomach may be simple overeating, especially with greasy and high-calorie food. Dogs will gulp down the food until their bowl is completely empty, so the power is basically in your hands.

To rule out overeating as a cause of digestion problems, try making smaller portions per meal and look for dog food for sensitive stomachs.

Switching from puppy to adult dog food, as well as changing brands, food type, or the feeding regimen can also be reasons for your dog's stomach aches.

Before making any abrupt changes in your dog's diet, consult a trusted vet and focus on gradual transitioning.

For example, instead of immediately switching from store-bought food to a raw dog diet, try combining the two or slowly introducing new ingredients.

How do I know my dog has digestive problems?

Asides from the apparent vomiting and diarrhea, you may notice other sickness symptoms, such as excessively licking of lips, gulping the air to fight the reflux, gaging or heaving, and even licking objects or paws. High temperature can be a sign of food poisoning, so watch out for dry and warm noses.

When feeling nauseated, dogs will sometimes eat grass to soothe the stomach or induce vomiting. In general, you will notice your pooch lying around, lacking energy and appetite.

Now let's explore some gentle herbal remedies that can help soothe your dog's stomach.

I. Slippery Elm

The inner bark of the slippery elm tree contains mucilage that coats, soothes, and protects the entire gastrointestinal tract when administered.

The mucilage helps reduce gastric inflammation and acidity, preventing or healing ulcers.

Slippery elm is effective for both constipation and diarrhea as it can add bulk to firm up loose stools or lubricate and soften to relieve straining.

For dogs, a typical dosage is 1/4 to 1 tsp powdered bark per 25 lbs body weight, stirred into food 1-3 times daily...

II. Marshmallow Root

Like slippery elm, marshmallow root contains mucilage that provides a protective barrier within the GI tract. The mucilage coats the stomach lining and esophagus to prevent ulcers.

Marshmallow root also reduces stomach acid secretion to relieve irritation. Its anti-inflammatory properties further soothe the gut lining.

For small dogs, 125mg powdered root can be given 1-2 times daily. Larger dogs can take 250-500mg daily.

Capsules are another option, with 1-2 given per day for smaller pets, 2-4 for large breeds. Give marshmallow root in a meal or with a treat to avoid choking on the powder.

III. Papaya

Papaya is a tropical fruit containing the proteolytic enzyme papain which substantially aids digestion. Papain breaks down proteins, fats, and carbohydrates for improved nutrient absorption. It also relieves constipation by softening stool. The antioxidants in papaya also reduce inflammation in the bowels.

For small dogs, give 1/3 to 1 tsp of mashed fresh papaya per 10 lbs body weight daily.

Large dogs can take 1-2 tbsp. Look for organic, fresh papaya and mash fully with no seeds. Capsules with papain enzyme are another option.

IV. Ginger

Ginger's active compounds called gingerols provide antinausea, antispasmodic, and gas-relieving effects, all helpful for digestive upsets. For dogs, 1/8 tsp per 20 lbs body weight of powdered ginger can be given twice daily when needed for nausea, vomiting, or gas.

For cats, just a pinch of ginger powder once a day is safe. Give ginger with meals for maximum soothing effects. Do not combine with blood thinners as it can increase anti-clotting effects. Reduce dosage if diarrhea develops.

V. Probiotics and Prebiotics

Supplementing pets with probiotics helps restore balance between healthy and harmful gut bacteria, especially after antibiotic use. Prebiotics provide "fuel" for probiotics.

Top probiotic strains for pets include Bifidobacterium, Lactobacillus, and Saccharomyces. Prebiotic fibers include inulin, fructooligosaccharides (FOS), and arabinogalactans. Quality pet supplements will contain research-backed strains. You can also give plain, unsweetened yogurt or kefir. Start with small amounts and monitor stool.

Summary

Below is a chart summarizing common digestive herbs, forms, and dosages:

Herb	Form	Dosage - Small Dogs	Dosage - Large Dogs
Slippery Elm	Powder	1/4-1 tsp per 25 lbs	1/2-1 tsp per 25 lbs
Marshmallo w Root	Powder, capsules	125mg	250-500mg
Ginger	Powder	1/8 tsp per 20 lbs	1/4 tsp per 20 lbs
Papaya	Fruit, enzyme caps	1/3-1 tsp per 10 lbs	1-2 tbsp per day

These digestive aids can help relieve nausea, vomiting, diarrhea, constipation, and other stomach issues in pets. Work with your vet to determine appropriate dosages and treatment duration.

VI. Lifestyle and Diet Changes

In addition to herbal supplementation, making certain lifestyle changes can further benefit your pet's digestion:

Dog Hydration and gastrointestinal problems

Symptoms like diarrhea and vomiting can be hazardous due to the sudden and excessive loss of body fluids.

Dehydration can further lead to serious health problems and require more intensive treatment if not treated properly.

Keeping your dog hydrated in these situations is essential; however, gulping water can make an already upset stomach even worse.

A simple trick you can try out is giving your dog ice chips or cubes in small amounts. The dog will slowly lick the ice, which will hydrate and refresh him.

Also, remove the water bowl out of reach and try giving a few spoonfuls of water from time to time.

Other tips:

- Feed a high quality, species-appropriate diet. Limit processed ingredients.
- Establish a consistent feeding routine and avoid sudden food changes.
- Ensure your pet drinks plenty of clean, fresh water to aid bowel health.
- Exercise daily to stimulate gut motility and prevent sluggish digestion.
- Schedule vet visits to rule out underlying disease if symptoms persist.

With some patience and the right mix of herbs, diet, and lifestyle adjustments, your pet's gastrointestinal system can get back on track for optimal health and comfort.

Chapter 4

Essential Oils for Flea, Tick and Skin Care

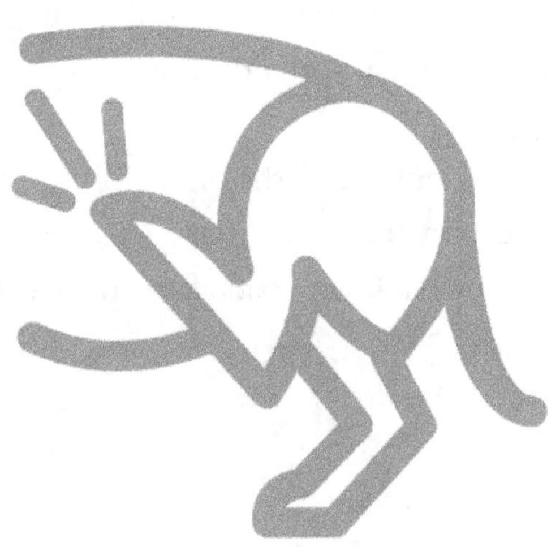

Like many pet owners, I dread the arrival of flea and tick season each year. My Labrador Retriever, Jamba, loves roaming our wooded trails and fields, which exposes her to these nasty parasites.

She's very sensitive and would scratch endlessly from just a few bites, chewing and licking herself raw. I tried every chemical-laden spray, shampoo, and collar from the pet store with limited success. The harsh pesticides also worried me. I wanted a natural, non-toxic way to repel fleas and ticks.

Then I discovered how using certain diluted essential oils can deter fleas, ticks, mosquitos and other insects while also benefiting skin and coat health. I can now protect Jamba with natural remedies I feel good about using on her and in our home.

One humid summer when the mosquitos were horrible, poor Jamba was getting bitten constantly on our walks. She'd obsessively gnaw at her paws and belly where they tended to bite most. I felt so guilty and panicked seeing the red, irritated skin and her distress.

That's when I quickly mixed up a natural bug spray with lavender, citronella, peppermint, and jojoba oil to mist onto her coat before going out. It worked wonderfully to repel the mosquitos without irritating her skin.

In this chapter, we'll explore proven essential oils that safely repel fleas, ticks, mosquitos and other pests when applied properly. I'll also share specific oil-based remedies to soothe common skin irritations, hot spots, ringworm, and more in pets. Using essential oils has made a huge difference in keeping Jamba comfortable during pest season and dealing with occasional skin issues.

Introduction

The Dangers of Fleas and Ticks

Fleas and ticks are frequent concerns for pet owners and can be extremely dangerous to dogs. They are parasites, meaning they take root in your dog's skin and suck blood and nutrients from the pup.

Fleas can consume up to 15 times their own body weight in blood, which can cause blood loss and anemia, especially in puppies. If a puppies' red blood cell count is depleted, it can be life-threatening. Some pets can also have an allergic reaction to fleas called flea allergy dermatitis.

Ticks can also cause blood loss and anemia, but even more dangerously, they carry diseases that can be deadly to your pet. Ticks can spread Lyme disease, which is a bacterial infection that can spread to dogs, cats, humans, and other mammals.

Symptoms of Lyme disease can include depression, swelling of the lymph nodes and joints, loss of appetite, fever, and even kidney failure.

If left untreated, flea and tick infestations can be deadly to dogs. Making sure to prevent and treat fleas and ticks ensures healthy pets that live long, happy lives.

I. Repelling Fleas and Ticks

Why Use Essential Oils?

When you take your dog to the vet for tick and flea control, they will probably prescribe either a medicated topical treatment or a preventative medication taken orally for tick and flea prevention.

Unfortunately, some of these medications have caused adverse neurological reactions in pets. Even if you don't notice the adverse effects right away, long-term or incorrect use of these products can cause skin irritation, vomiting, or respiratory problems.

With continued use of these products, fleas can eventually develop immunity to them, and they'll no longer be effective in protecting against flea infestations.

The use of essential oils is a great alternative to oral and topical medications because they're all-natural and can be made right at home, so you know exactly what goes into them. They are pet safe when used in the right quantities and applications, and they can even provide added benefits, like providing antiseptic properties to help heal flea and tick bites and soothing itchy, irritated skin.

Essential oils offer a variety of health benefits to humans, and when used correctly, they can provide the same for your pets.

<u>As a general rule of thumb</u>, do not use essential oils on your pet in any way you wouldn't use them on yourself. Essential oils are extremely potent and can cause irritation, itchiness, redness, and other side effects when applied undiluted.

It is important to always use carrier oil to dilute essential oils before applying them to your pet's skin. A carrier oil is a neutral, plant-based oil that is safe for the skin in large quantities and is necessary for dilution. Examples of pet-safe carrier oils are:

Coconut Oil
Aloe Vera Oil
Avocado Oil
Sunflower Oil
Sweet Almond Oil
Castor Oil
Jojoba Oil

Make sure to learn the warning signs of essential oil toxicity in dogs. If you notice your pet experiencing vomiting, diarrhea, wobbliness, excessive drooling, depression, lethargy, weakness, tremors, or any other abnormal behavior, stop treatment immediately and consult your veterinarian.

Certain essential oils contain compounds that naturally deter or even kill fleas, ticks, mosquitos and other pests through toxicity or scent-based repellency:

Peppermint Oil – The menthol in peppermint oil drives away fleas, ticks, mosquitos, mites and lice. It can be diluted in a spray or added to pet shampoo. Do not apply undiluted.

Cedarwood Oil – Has a strong scent that repels fleas and ticks. Also acts as an insecticide. Can be diluted and applied to pet bedding.

Citronella Oil – Repels mosquitos, fleas and ticks with its strong lemon-like aroma. Often used in candles and sprays. Needs heavy dilution on pets.

Lemongrass Oil – Contains citronellal that repels fleas and ticks. Provides lasting effects when applied properly to coats.

Lavender Oil – Its scent deters fleas and ticks while also calming pets. Dilute and apply to coat or pet bedding.

Eucalyptus Oil – Repels ticks and can be diluted in spray formulas. Has some insecticidal effects against parasites.

II. Treating Skin Irritations

Dogs and cats can suffer from dry, itchy skin or develop hot spots and infections from excessive licking and scratching. This can result from allergies, insect bites, underlying conditions or sensitivities to products. Essential oils can provide soothing relief when properly diluted based on the pet and condition:

Lavender Oil – Soothes allergy symptoms and skin irritations. Calms itching and supports healing of damaged skin.

Tea Tree Oil - Has antifungal, antimicrobial properties to fight infections causing itching and hot spots. Also reduces inflammation.

Chamomile Oil – Calms skin irritations and allergy symptoms thanks to its antihistamine effects. Speeds healing.

Basil Oil – Contains antibacterial compounds to treat hot spots, wounds. Also acts as an insect repellent.

Marjoram Oil – Relieves inflammation and pruritis causing itchy skin allergies in pets. Calms reactive skin.

Aloe Vera Gel – The perfect soothing carrier for distressed skin. Combine with lavender, tea tree for homemade remedy.

III. Fighting Ringworm and Other Fungi

Ringworm is a highly contagious fungal skin infection in pets often passed from contact with an infected animal or environment. Some essential oils contain antifungal compounds and can be applied topically to treat ringworm in pets when properly diluted:

Oregano Oil - Shown to inhibit growth of ringworm more effectively than prescription antifungals. Dilute before applying.

Thyme Oil – Contains thymol that disrupts fungal cell membranes. Apply diluted on cotton pad directly to affected areas.

Tea Tree Oil – Studies demonstrate anti-fungal effects against ringworm. Dilute in carrier oil or shampoo.

Turmeric Oil - Curcumin has antifungal properties that may help clear ringworm. Can be taken orally in food.

These oils should never be given internally/orally. Monitor for skin sensitivity when treating fungal infections. Seek vet care if infection worsens.

IV. How to Use Essential Oils on Dogs

There are a variety of effective ways you can use essential oils to repel and kill fleas and ticks on dogs. Different methods will be most effective for different oils.

Mix With Shampoo

A great way to easily apply essential oils directly to your dog's skin without causing irritation is to mix it with their regular shampoo during bath time. Adding 5-10 drops of essential oil to your dog's shampoo while bathing is a great, all-natural way to make sure pests stay away. This method works well with lavender oil, neem oil, and rosemary oil.

Diffuse It

Diffusing essential oils is a great way to spread their healing properties throughout your entire home. By placing natural pest repellent oils in your diffuser, you can kill and repel any pests in your home, not just the ones that have already rooted into your dog's fur. We recommend diffusing lemongrass oil, cedar oil, and lavender oil.

Make A Spray

Mixing essential oils with water in a spray bottle is a great no-fuss way to keep fleas and ticks away. Simply 5-10 drops of undiluted essential oil with 8 oz. of water and place it in an empty spray bottle. Then, simply spray your dog's coat with the mixture a few times per week. This method works well with lemongrass oil and rosemary oil.

Apply To Skin

The easiest way to apply essential oils to your dog's fur is to simply place a few drops on them in key areas (mixed with a carrier oil, of course). You can place a few drops of diluted essential oil under your dog's collar, behind their shoulder blades, or at the base of their tail. This works best with rose geranium oil, neem oil, lavender oil, and clove oil.

While some essential oils can be used undiluted for things like cleaning, oils should always be diluted when applied directly to pets' skin or coat.

The general guideline is 0.5-1% solution for small animals.

Carrier Oils – Coconut, olive, jojoba, almond and other carrier oils help evenly distribute and dilute essential oils for safe topical use.

Mixing Tips – Add just a few drops of essential oils per ounce of shampoo or water. Shake sprays well before each use.

Storage – Store unused mixtures in dark bottles in a cool area to preserve potency and shelf life.

Precautions – Test mixtures on a small skin area first. Rinse immediately if irritation occurs. Keep treatments out of eyes, ears, and mouth.

V. Sample Recipes

Flea and Tick Collar:
Add 5 drops each of lavender, peppermint, cedarwood, lemongrass and citronella oils to 1 Tbsp of a carrier oil like coconut or jojoba oil. Apply a few drops around your pet's collar. Reapply weekly.

Soothing Skin Gel:
Combine 1/4 cup aloe vera gel with 5 drops lavender oil and 5 drops tea tree oil. Apply sparingly to affected areas 1-2 times a day after bathing and air drying your pet's coat.

Antifungal Shampoo:
In 1 cup gentle, unscented pet shampoo, add 3 drops oregano oil, 3 drops thyme oil, and 5 drops tea tree oil. Lather onto the pet and let sit for 5 minutes before rinsing thoroughly.

Calming Bed Spritz:
Add 10 drops of lavender oil and 5 drops of marjoram oil to 2 ounces of water in a spray bottle.

Lightly mist your pet's bedding to create a soothing atmosphere.

Using essential oils safely and effectively can support your pet's health and comfort in many ways. But they should never replace veterinary care when needed. Consult your vet if skin issues worsen or persist. Let's continue exploring the aromatherapy benefits for our furry friends!

Chapter 5

Herbs for Immunity and Liver Support

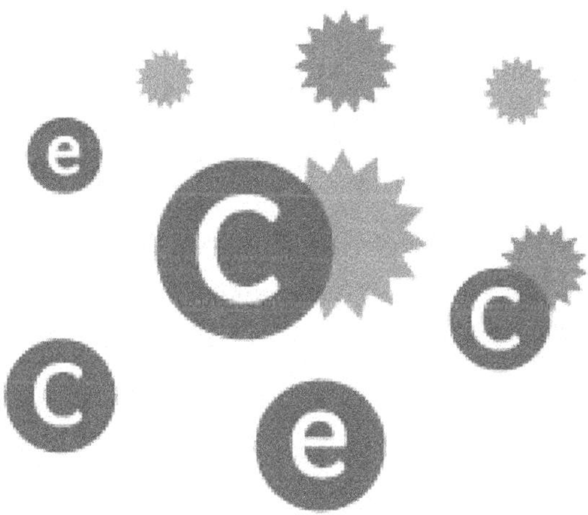

Introduction

A properly functioning immune system and healthy liver are vital to a pet's wellbeing and longevity. The immune system acts as the body's defense against viruses, bacteria, and disease. A strong immunity prevents chronic inflammation and fights infection.

The liver filters toxins and produces proteins essential for blood clotting and other vital functions. Over time, issues like chronic illness, toxins, and certain medications can tax these important systems. Herbal remedies can provide gentle, effective support.

I like to incorporate herbs for immunity and liver health as part of Jamba's preventative care routine. During times of stress, traveling, or potential exposure to illness, I increase her supplementation as added protection.

Certain herbs help regulate immune response, while others provide antioxidants and anti-inflammatory benefits. Some aid natural detoxification abilities of the liver and kidneys. Let's explore the top herbs for bolstering these critical systems in pets.

What is Natural and Herbal Liver Support?

A dog's liver is an extremely important part of the digestive and immune systems, filtering out toxins ingested by the animal and preventing them from being absorbed into the blood.

However, certain health conditions can result in the liver starting to malfunction and thereby release quantities of these toxins into the body. In extreme cases, the liver will stop functioning altogether, allowing extremely hazardous substances to build up in the tissues of the dog's vital organs.

In order to stop this from happening, a vet can provide various pharmaceutical drugs to counteract the effects of the condition in question.

However, this treatment can be accompanied with careful dietary supplementation to help keep the liver in a good condition.

Natural products containing things such as antioxidants can be a great way to both combat and prevent liver problems.

I. Echinacea

Echinacea is one of the most researched herbs for enhancing immune response in humans and animals. Compounds like polysaccharides activate beneficial immune cells that destroy invading pathogens.

Other compounds have antiviral effects against common viruses. Studies indicate short term use of Echinacea can help prevent and treat upper respiratory infections in dogs.

For small dogs, 250mg daily is a typical dose, while larger breeds can take 500-1000mg per day, split into two doses. Tinctures, powders, and whole plant products are available. It's best used for up to two weeks at a time, with breaks in between.

II. Astragalus

Astragalus is an excellent adaptogenic herb traditionally used in Chinese medicine to modulate and strengthen the entire immune system.

It appears to stimulate underactive immune activity while damping overactivity and inflammation.

Astragalus also helps combat cancer and kidney disease in dogs and cats according to some studies.

Pairing it with reishi mushroom may boost effects. Use 100-500mg powdered root per day for dogs based on size, 100mg cats. Best given daily for 2-4 weeks.

III. Milk Thistle

Milk thistle is one of the most validated herbs for supporting liver function and health. Its active compounds called silymarins protect liver cells from toxins and damage while aiding regeneration.

It's been used to treat liver disease, cancer, kidney problems in dogs and cats.

For small dogs, 125mg milk thistle capsules or extract can be given daily.

Large dogs can take 250-500mg per day. Look for products standardized to 80% silymarins for best effects.

Milk thistle can be used long term without harm

V. Dandelion

The roots and leaves of common dandelion are a potent medicinal. Dandelion improves bile flow to help remove toxins from the liver, while also gently diuretic to reduce strain on kidneys.

The bitters support digestive health. Dose is 1/8-1/4 tsp powdered leaf per 10lbs weight once daily. Capsules with 500mg extracts are also available.

Monitor for increased urination and bowel movements. Best used for 2-4 week intervals.

VI. Reishi and Turkey Tail Mushrooms

Medicinal mushrooms like reishi and turkey tail are adaptogens that balance and strengthen immune response.

They have been shown in research to fight cancer and viruses in pets. Turkey tail also aids digestion.

These medicinal mushrooms contain polysaccharides, antioxidants, and other immune-enhancing compounds.

Give 100mg powder, 500mg capsules, or 5 drops extract/tincture daily. Can be rotated with other herbs or given short term.

Below is a summary chart of key immunity and liver herbs, their forms, and dosage ranges:

Herb	Form	Dosage Range - Dogs	Dosage Range - Cats
Echinacea	Capsules, tincture, dried herb	250-1000 mg	100-300 mg
Milk Thistle	Capsules, extract	125-500 mg	50-200 mg
Astragalus	Powder	100-1000 mg	100-300 mg
Dandelion	Dried leaf, capsules	1/8-1/2 tsp per 10 lbs	1/8 tsp

VII. Lifestyle Support

Some additional tips to keep your pet's immunity and liver function optimal:

- Feed species-appropriate, antioxidant-rich whole foods diet
- Avoid unnecessary vaccinations/drugs that strain the liver
- Use natural flea/tick prevention methods
- Minimize environmental and food toxins
- Manage stress through training, routines, pheromones
- Visit integrative vet for diagnostics when needed

Supporting your pet's vital systems boosts their health, wellbeing and longevity. Consult your vet before using herbs, especially with pets who have medical conditions or take other medications. Let's continue exploring safe, natural ways to care for our furry companions!

Conclusion

Summary

We've covered a lot of ground exploring gentle, effective herbal remedies for common health issues in pets.

We discussed herbs that can provide relief for chronic joint pain and arthritis, such as turmeric, CBD, and boswellia. Valerian, chamomile, and other calming herbs offer natural support for anxious pets without sedating side effects.

For digestion issues, slippery elm, marshmallow root, and papaya can soothe upset stomachs and restore gut health. Essential oils like lavender and tee tree make safe, natural solutions for flea, tick, and skin problems.

And we reviewed immunity and liver herbs like echinacea, milk thistle and reishi mushrooms for whole body wellness.

The major takeaway is pets can benefit immensely from natural supplements just as we do. Herbs allow us to address our furry companions' health concerns gently, without necessarily having to resort quickly to strong prescription medications.

Of course herbs are not replacements for qualified veterinary guidance and care. But used wisely, they can be wonderful complements to promote comfort, vitality and quality of life.

I've seen amazing improvements first-hand in my Labrador Retriever Jamba since incorporating more herbal remedies.

I. Importance of Vet Guidance

While I'm a big believer in the power of herbs, they should never be used in place of proper veterinary care and oversight. Partnering with a holistic or integrative vet knowledgeable about complementary therapies is ideal. Such vets look at the whole patient while being open to gentle, natural treatment options along with conventional care as needed. Some standard diagnostics I recommend are:

- Bloodwork to check for issues like kidney/liver disease, diabetes, thyroid problems
- Stool analysis to rule out parasites or pathogenic bacteria
- Skin scrapings to diagnose allergies or fungal infections

- X-rays and joint fluid analysis for orthopedic problems
- Ultrasound to visualize abdominal issues or growths

Getting to the root cause allows appropriate treatment. Herbs can then provide adjunct support based on your trusted vet's guidance.

II. Dosing and Safety

When first using herbal supplements with your pet, always start slowly and observe how they respond:

- Give smaller doses at first and work up to target dosages
- Look for any unusual reactions like digestive upset or drowsiness
- Adjust dosage down if negative response and consult your vet
- Ensure proper dosage for pet's size - don't exceed guidelines
- Rotate herbs to avoid overtaxing organs like the liver

Only purchase high quality pet supplements from reputable manufacturers. Never give your pet herbs intended for human consumption, as dosing differs. With sensible precautions, herbal remedies can be very safe and beneficial.

III. Sourcing Quality Herbs

As the pet supplement industry is still lightly regulated, procuring high quality products is essential. Seek companies with extensive in-house testing for potency, purity and safety.

It's worth contacting manufacturers to ask questions and request certificates of analysis. Organically grown, non-GMO, responsibly wild-harvested herbs are ideal.

Buying in small quantities and refrigerating after opening preserves freshness.

IV. Final Thoughts

It's been a pleasure to share my passion for improving pet's lives holistically.

I hope this book provides you with many natural options to explore for your furry friends' wellbeing. Please don't hesitate to consult me with any questions you may have along your journey.

I always love hearing success stories and feedback from fellow pet lovers as we learn together.

Most importantly, trust your intuition - you know your pets better than anyone.

Let's continue honoring the animals who bring us such joy by providing the gentlest care possible.

To our pets' good health!